How To Lose Weight Fast In 10 Days

I0844216

AN AMAZING WEIGHT LOSS GUIDE

TO ACHIEVE A FLAT TUMMY, A HOT BODY IN GOOD SHAPE THAT YOU'LL LOVE WITH LESS TIME AND WITHOUT EXERCISE, ALL IN 2 WEEKS!

By Stella Perrine

Copyright©2022 Stella Perrine

All Rights Reserved.

<u>**TABLE OF CONTENTS**</u>

<u>**INTRODUCTION**</u>

<u>**CHAPTER ONE**</u>

General knowledge on fat burners as a whole.

<u>**CHAPTER TWO**</u>

The ingredients in a fat burner supplement.

<u>**CHAPTER THREE**</u>

How this miracle pill was invented.

<u>**CHAPTER FOUR**</u>

The miracle pill: express fat burner.

<u>**CHAPTER FIVE**</u>

Why you must have the new fat burner express (ultra clean premium detox).

<u>**EXTRAS**</u>

INTRODUCTION

This book is for everybody keen on losing weight independently old enough.

Have you at any point asked why losing such a lot of weight is generally so troublesome? Quit enduring yourself and trench calorie counting, yoyo eats less carbs and inordinate activity for good.

Indeed, it's still truly conceivable to accomplish your fantasy body this mid year, spring or whatever the season.

The most effective method; *How to lose weight in 10 days* is an astounding book that shows us how to lose weight without working out, while never going to the rec center, no active work and stress while you eat anything you desire.

Everybody battling with corpulence and weight reduction issues needs this book at the present time.

CHAPTER ONE

General knowledge on fat burners as a whole.

What are Fat Terminators?

Fat burners, killers, eliminators or terminators as the name suggests are drugs that assist in weight reduction by wearing out fat subsequently decreasing the amount of fat.

How really does fat terminator Function in the body?

Fat eliminators work by hoisting your circulatory strain and expanding your general energy use which may ultimately prompt weight reduction additional time. In any case, it is prudent you play it safe assuming that you are taking drugs or as of now have hypertension.

What are Fat Eliminator Enhancements?

Fat Killers supplements work by expanding your resting metabolic rate. The active ingredients present help to get rid of the body fat.

Do Fat terminator supplements work?

Fat terminator supplements work by hoisting your pulse and your general energy use.
 They work by:
-Expanding your digestion.
-Lessening how much fat your body ingests. Furthermore;
-Smothering your hunger.

Are Fat Terminator supplements safe?

You can not actually determine what is contained in a fat terminator pill or case; since certain fixings are not recorded on the container.

A portion of these dynamic fixings can cause:
1.) Tension,
2.) Liver issues,
3.) Expanded Pulse And;
4.) Heart issues.
 Prior to taking these enhancements, counsel your primary care physician first.

CHAPTER TWO

The ingredients in a fat burner supplement.

To the extent that we realize fat terminators are taken orally either in a case or tablet structure.

Be that as it may, what are the fixings in a fat terminator supplement?

They contain various nutrients, fiber and caffeine, minerals, spices and different plants.

1.) Caffeine:

Caffeine is a typical fixing obtained from cocoa. It works by animating the sensory system in this manner consuming calories. Caffeine can be seen as in: Espresso, tea or chocolate.

2.) Yohimbe:

Yohimbe is a plant compound that comes from the bark of an evergreen tree. It is normal in fat eliminator supplements however it likewise has adverse consequences. For example,

-Tumult;

-Tension;
-Expanded Circulatory strain and;
-Heart issues.

3.) Green Tea Concentrate:

Green tea helps consume calories and diminish the sum of how much fat you assimilate from food.

4.) Solvent Fiber:

This specific fixing is not tracked down a lot in every single fat killer. Dissolvable Fiber forestalls/control your body from retaining fat from food.

5.) Vitamin B-complex:

They help by using sugars, fats and proteins to put away energy as opposed to allowing it to go to fat.

CHAPTER THREE

How this miracle pill was invented.

The name of this miracle pill is called **EXPRESS FAT BURNER** and this is the way it was imagined.

A misfortune in her family made Dr. Olayinka understand that eating regimens, actual work, and tablets as well as liposuction are hazardous to wellbeing to some extent in the cases and they don't take care of the issue of overabundance weight.

What roused Dr. Olayinka is simply private as it comes from an exceptionally private encounter.

Barely a long time back, her mom passed on from hypertension, she had been overweight for a long time. Despite the fact that She was fine, and her mother had been on a strict diet and had drilled high impact exercise for a very long time she had been attempting to free weight for some time now, however after a second a stroke killed her in her rest. Her grandma likewise passed on for a similar explanation.

Dr. Olayinka began concentrating after her demise to comprehend the issues associated with excess weight and how to address them. She was stunned, after understanding that weight control plans, active work, and pills as well as liposuction are half perilous for wellbeing and don't actually take care of the issue.

During the past three years she examined and zeroed in on this issue a great deal. That is the new strategy to fix the weight reduction issues that everybody's discussing now, a technique that emerged while she was thinking of her postulation.

Olayinka was offered millions in various monetary standards including dollars and euros for her earth shattering development. Yet, she benevolently declined.

What an insightful choice since weight reduction items are extravagant and most times far off for the everyday person.

With Dr. Olayinka's cutting edge it won't just impact the world overall however it will presently be accessible for the average person at a reasonable cost. Well that is a marvel!

CHAPTER FOUR

The miracle pill: express fat burner.

What is an Express Fat terminator?

Express Fat Burner premium is a capsule which is a characteristic enhancement which helps in weight reduction to give an alluring body with everything looking great.

What is crafted by Express Fat killer?

Crafted by express fat terminator is to wear out fat, tone muscles, assemble shape and bring out curves.

How In all actuality does Fat Eliminator Premium work in the body?

The readiness was made in view of Olayinka's thought. It contains cell reinforcements that give signs to a particular part of the cerebrum that is the amygdala to quit absorbing calories, greasy layers and remove the longing for unhealthy food. It was termed or identified as the **"ULTRA CLEAN PREMIUM DETOX"**

Ultra clean premium Detox is a readiness that should be taken for treatment stringently with headings. It contains 25 concentrates, thereby making the fat consuming cycle sped up by multiple times.

It speeds up the digestion and restores the craft by the endocrine framework, invigorates tissue recovery and has marvelous impacts for the decrease of craving.

CHAPTER FIVE

Why you must have the new fat burner express (ultra clean premium detox).

In this last section of this book, I might want to discuss why anybody battling with corpulence or anybody who truly needs to shed off weight or perhaps knows somebody who needs this supernatural occurrence pill ought to get it now!

Here, I will uncover the advantages and why you needn't bother with some other weight reduction pills in your day to day existence once more. Just EXPRESS FAT BURNER.

1.) No secondary effects:
The fundamental and most significant thing in a fat eliminator is it ought to Make NO SIDE Impacts. As examined before, incidental effects could go from tumults to liver issues.

Something wonderful about this item is that it makes no side impacts! Indeed! Envision accomplishing your fantasy objective without really any feeling of dread toward secondary effects over the long haul. Now that is actually a blessing from heaven!

2.) Say a Colossal bye to consuming less calories:

Eating fewer carbs will doubtlessly be a relic of times gone by with Dr. Olayinka's most recent creation.

3.) No pressure, Less time and bounty Gain:

With the Ultra Clean premium Detox, Subcutaneous fat and trouble spots vanish everlastingly at a pace of 500grams each day with no pressure or active work like going to the exercise center.

4.) Reasonable:

Indeed, it's exceptionally simple to snatch for you, for myself and for everyone at an entirely reasonable cost.

EXTRAS

Cost

The Express fat terminator is sold at around 47.02 US dollars.

Directions

Take 1-3 pills before dinners with a glass of water.

Pls counsel your PCP first and get endorsed on this medication first with the sufficient measure of pills to take.

So why not attempt this marvel pill and watch your life altering event for eternity. Here are a few declarations of individuals who have utilized this marvel pill:

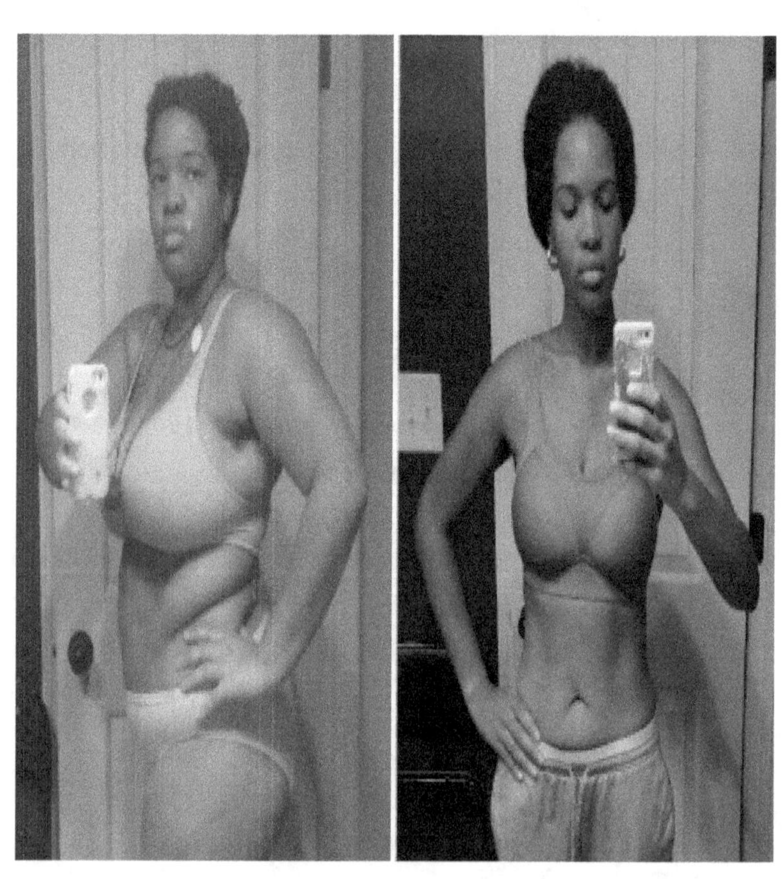

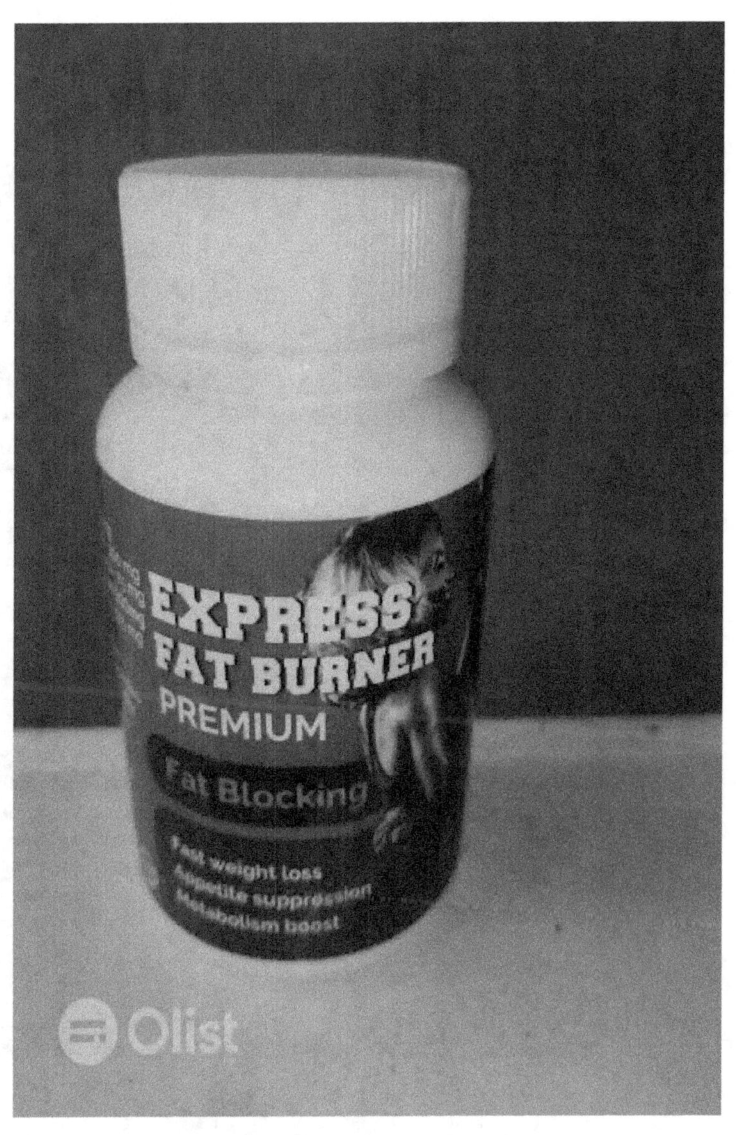
EXPRESS
FAT BURNER
PREMIUM
Fat Blocking
Fast weight loss
Appetite suppression
Metabolism boost
Olist

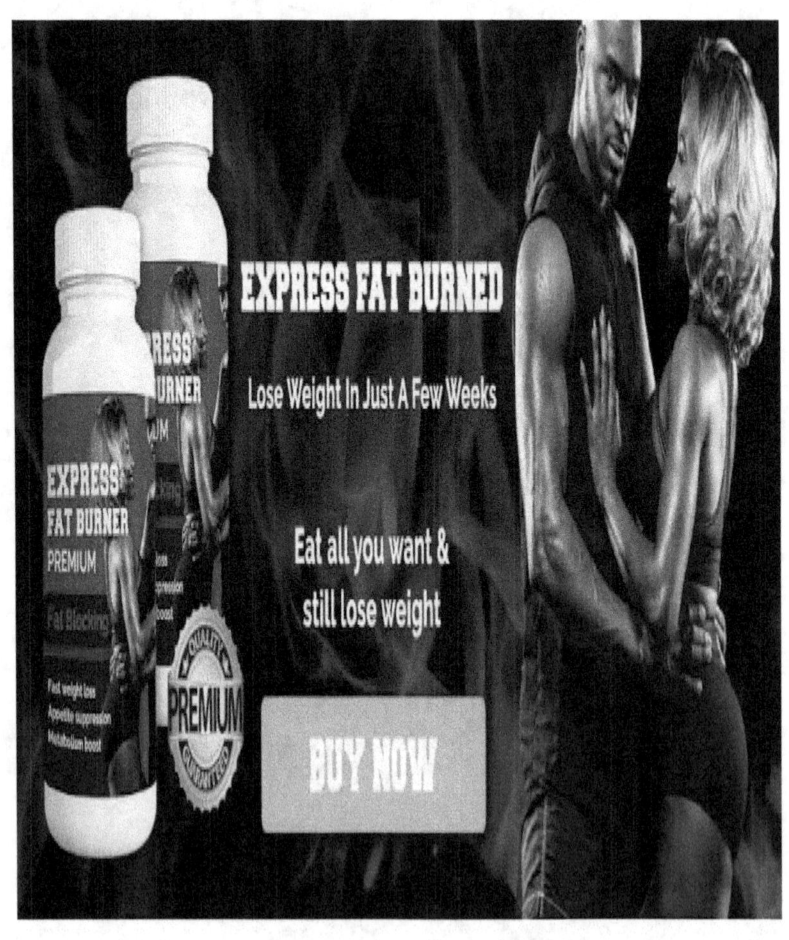
EXPRESS FAT BURNED
Lose Weight In Just A Few Weeks
Eat all you want &
still lose weight
BUY NOW
EXPRESS
FAT BURNER
PREMIUM
Fast weight loss
Appetite suppression
Metabolism boost
PREMIUM
QUALITY GUARANTEED

Pls do well to leave positive reviews on this book.